THE FOUNTAIN OF YOUTH & ETERNAL HEALTH

By - Laleh Shaban M.D.
Michael Scalise C.H.C.

Published September, 2017
Copyright 2017

ISBN-13: 978-1977820891
ISBN-10: 1977820891

ACKNOWLEDGEMENTS

I want to thank my wonderful husband, Michael, my son, Arian, and my daughter, Nina, for always supporting me. I want to also thank Mrs. Rebecca Jones for being extremely supportive. I would also like to acknowledge and extend a grateful "thank you" to everyone who has helped me write this book, including Mr. Clint Arthur, Ms. Ali Savage, Maryann King, and my wonderful friend, Fariba, and her family. I am grateful to have a job that I love along with wonderful patients and staff.

On the cover of this book is my daughter, Nina. When she was 13 months old, she came down with a severe case of pneumonia. We were sitting in her hospital room on a chair next to her crib. The nurse had kneeled down and was pushing a medicine into my daughter's PICC line. Within seconds, my daughter made a funny noise and lost her body's tone; she had had an adverse reaction to the medicine. I looked at her and she was blue. I knew my baby had died in my arms. I looked at the nurse and she screamed, "What do we do?" I yelled, "Call the code." Then I threw my daughter in her crib and began to run her code. I ran that code with every breath I had. I was like a lioness protecting her cub. After 50 long seconds she began to cry. It was the most joyful moment of my life. Today she is 22 years old and healthy. I feel so blessed to have her and the rest of my family in my life. We live this life once, so let's take care of ourselves the best we can.

Introduction

People have been searching for the fountain of youth since 1521 when Ponce de Leon, a Spanish explorer, discovered what he thought was the fountain of youth but in actuality it was Florida.

I have been practicing Functional Medicine for over five years. Functional medicine is the future of medicine. It seeks to uncover the root causes of diseases, and to treat the whole body and not just a symptom. More and more patients are fed up with being handed a pill, because they know it doesn't cure their problem.

According to Zion Market Research Global Report, the cost of anti-aging remedies and cures were valued at 140 billion dollars in 2015 and is estimated to reach 216 billion dollars in 2021. These remedies include everything from balancing hormones, oxidative therapies, aesthetic procedures, weight loss programs, body sculpting and genital rejuvenation for both men and women, and more.

What is aging? There are many different theories of aging. One theory is the telomere theory. Telomeres are caps on the end strands of DNA within our cells. Every time a cell replicates, a tiny bit of the telomere falls off. Think of them like the hard plastic tips on a shoelace that prevents the shoelace from fraying. Once all the telomere is gone, a cell can no longer replicate. It is believed that most human cells can only replicate about 50 times. Once enough cells die off in an organ, there will be organ failure and death.

A second theory of aging is the endocrine theory. The endocrine system is your hormone system. Hormones are chemicals that are produced in one organ, but send signals to other organs via the blood stream. Conventional doctors will tell you that as you age your hormones decline. A functional medicine doctor will tell you that you age **because** your hormones decline. Every physical sign of aging is a hormone deficiency. If you restore your hormones to youthful levels, you will look and feel younger. Restoring hormones is a critical tool for a functional medicine physician in order to prevent premature death.

A third theory of aging is the gastrointestinal (GI) theory. You have your outside skin and your inside skin. Your GI tract is your inside skin, and is your interface between the outside world and your blood. It is protected by a layer of cells one-cell thick, and if spread out, would cover the area the size of a tennis court. For your body to function, you must be able to obtain nutrients from your food. By age 60, almost half of Americans have inadequate stomach acid, which is necessary to digest protein and absorb minerals from food. So, even though people eat enough food, they are malnourished from digestion problems, which in turn leads to chronic illnesses. Ninety-eight percent of Americans have at least one nutrient deficiency, and most have numerous deficiencies, which lead to chronic illnesses and weight gain.

I've heard many doctors claim that our modern healthcare system has greatly improved the lifespan of Americans. Before we explain about life expectancy, we should explain what it really means. Life expectancy is a statistical measure of the average time someone is expected to live. It is usually expressed as life expectancy at birth. That is one of the most misleading statistics. If someone is quoting life expectancy at birth, they are probably trying to deceive you. For example, if the life expectancy at birth was 40 years of age, it does not mean that most people died at age 40. Most would have died before the age of 20 or older than the age of 55. Suppose you had two children, one who died at age 5, and one at age 75. Their average life expectancy would be 40, even though neither of them died near 40.

Historically, many children never reached adulthood. Typically from one-third to one-half of children died of some childhood disease. This greatly throws off average life expectancy from birth. A much more meaningful statistic is the life expectancy of a 25 year-old, or a 65-year old.

In ancient Rome, a 65-year-old had a life expectancy of 72. In 1900, a white male at the age of 65 had a life expectancy of 77 years. So, in 2,000 years, the life expectancy of a 65-year-old increased by only five years. By the year 2000, the life expectancy of a 65-year-old white male was 81 years. So, a person could make the claim that in the last one hundred years, modern medicine has increased a 65-year-old's life expectancy by four years, but that too is likely misleading.

We know that wealth plays a very strong role in life expectancy. Poor people die sooner than wealthy people, and there has been a significant increase in wealth in the last one hundred years. The availability of food has vastly improved, and the cost dropped considerably. Modern medicine has made tremendous improvements in preventing childhood deaths, but has done very poorly in preventing deaths from heart disease and cancer. Startlingly, the third leading cause of death is medical mistakes, so modern healthcare can be dangerous.

Aging and premature deaths are two distinct concepts. To live a long life, you can't die prematurely from a condition that is preventable. One hundred years ago, the typical causes of death were from conditions such as bacterial and viral infections. Heart disease and cancer were relatively rare; now they are the top two reasons why we die prematurely.

There are many controversies and thoughts about whether the fountain of youth is real. As a medical doctor specializing in geriatrics, nutrition and antiaging medicine, I say the fountain of youth is real. But if you want to find it, you have to look inside your own body. So how do you access the fountain of youth? Well, there are seven basic steps you need to take to access the fountain of youth inside your own body. The remainder of this book will discuss these seven steps.

TABLE OF CONTENTS

Acknowledgements..iii

Introduction.. v

Chapter One
Step 1
Don't trust your doctor............................. 1

Chapter Two
Step 2
Think positive..................................... 13

Chapter Three
Step 3
Balancing Your Hormones........................... 21

Chapter Four
Step 4
Biotransformation (Detoxification)................. 39

Chapter Five
Step 5
Life Style Changes 49

Chapter Six
Step 6

Sleep 67

Chapter Seven
Step 7
Stress 81

Chapter Eight
Platelet rich plasma joint and soft tissue injections 87

Chapter One

✣ STEP 1 ✣

DON'T TRUST YOUR DOCTOR

You should not blindly trust your physician or healthcare providers. Why? Because the third-leading cause of death in the USA appears to be medical errors. Conservatively the actual number of deaths from medical errors is at least 251,000 per year. **10% of all deaths are now due to medical error**, and medical errors are an under-recognized cause of death because they are not reported and tracked by the Centers for Disease Control (CDC.) This data was released in 2016 by researchers from Johns Hopkins Medical Center. In 2013, the CDC reported the top three causes of death in the U.S. were heart disease (611,105), cancer (584,881), and chronic respiratory disease (149,205), but since medical errors are not tracked by the CDC, they should be in third place.

When my patients challenge me, I like it. Doctors are not gods. We live in a world where we have access to information and it can be done by pushing a button on your phone or computer. There are also books, journals, webinars and seminars that can support your own research. Doctors have been pressured to see as many patients per day as possible in order to keep their offices open. With poor reimbursements from insurance companies, doctors are often forced financially to see over 40 patients a day; this does not include all the urgent incoming calls, addressing abnormal stat reports, or having emergency situations at the office which were not anticipated.

As a result of this pressure, many physicians are spending five minutes with each patient and only addressing one health complaint in that amount of time. What happens if a patient has more than one health complaint? They will have to make another appointment which may require a two-or-three-month wait, simply to return for the second complaint (let's hope the second complaint wasn't a symptom of a serious condition such as a heart attack, stroke, organ damage, severe infection, etc.). This invariably will cause the patient to end up utilizing the hospital emergency room or die due to failure to get the appropriate medical attention. This could be you or your loved ones.

Physicians are constantly overwhelmed and under time constraints and end up regularly missing out on their lunch breaks. In lieu of having a full lunch, they snack on whatever is quick and easy, becoming unhealthy, oftentimes becoming quite ill themselves. Recent studies show that the number one cause of death in doctors-in-training used to be suicide, but currently is now cancer.

Some physicians will hire mid-levels such as physician assistants or nurse practitioners to see patients which can be either helpful or harmful depending on the mid-level's personality, training, experience, and knowledge. As a result, questioning your physician or any of your health care providers can eliminate medical mistakes that can cost you your health, and/or your life.

I personally encourage my patients to always read not just the information provided to them by my practice, but to research it from alternate sources. Becoming knowledgeable about your own health condition will move you to be in the captain's position of your own ship, and you can lead the way to a healthier life. You should always seek a second or even a third opinion once you are diagnosed with a condition and given a treatment plan.

Mainstream physicians, also known as conventional physicians, are doctors that have attended medical school and residency programs at various hospitals with different trainings. As a physician who practiced mainstream medicine for 15 years, I can tell you that what you learn is all based on pharmaceutical influences. The only tool a conventional physician can use to treat a disease, is a prescription drug. I now practice Functional Medicine, which seeks to find the root cause of the disease or condition, and try to get patients off their prescription drugs.

In twelve years of training, I had only one hour of nutritional education, and that was mainly on the diabetic diet; even that dietary education is not valid in the functional medicine world.

This is an example of what is wrong with mainstream medicine.

The CDC released a report in 2017 stating that 100 million Americans are diabetic or pre-diabetic. For those over age 65, nearly one-half are diabetic or pre-diabetic. But the blood tests they used are not early detection markers for diabetes. They used fasting glucose and Hemoglobin A1c (HbA1c), but these tests do not indicate elevated glucose until you have already lost about 70-80% of your pancreatic function. We use the very earliest markers for detecting diabetes, and we detect the disease decades before fasting glucose and HbA1c become elevated. From the tests we perform, the real number of adult Americans that are pre-diabetic or diabetic is closer to 80%.

Diabetes is caused from Insulin Resistance. Insulin Resistance is synonymous with Metabolic Syndrome (aka Syndrome X). Metabolic syndrome is a cluster of diseases such as hypertension, heart disease, diabetes, obesity, Alzheimer's, stroke, many cancers, and gout. In other words, most of the chronic illnesses that Americans will die from, are due to Insulin Resistance.

4

The first detectable signs of prediabetes in a blood test is a decline in a hormone called adiponectin, and rise in α-hydroxybutyrate and a decline in Linoleoyl-GPC. The next blood marker to rise is proinsulin. This is the precursor to make insulin, and indicates that your body has been under pressure to make too much insulin, even though the fasting insulin level appears to be normal. Then insulin will eventually begin to rise, and after it stays elevated, only then will fasting glucose and HbA1c begin to rise. At this point, your pancreatic beta cells are 70-80% damaged and cannot create enough insulin to keep blood sugar under control.

An ideal HbA1c is from 4.4 to 5.2. When HbA1c is above 5.2, you are at increased risk for diabetes, heart disease, many cancers and Alzheimer's, and have more brain shrinkage as you age. An HbA1c above 6.5 is considered diabetic, and from 5.7 to 6.4 is considered pre-diabetic. An optimal fasting glucose level would be from 75 to 86 mg/dl, even though 70-100 mg/dl is currently considered the "normal" lab ranges for glucose.

Diet is the most powerful treatment for most chronic conditions; this is especially true for diabetes and insulin resistance. To learn that your doctor's training regarding the most effective cure for your health has been one hour in their 12 years of training should scare you enough to want to be proactive and learn more about the condition and proper upkeep of your health. Mainstream physicians have been taught to use medication as the main course of therapy.

Medication only addresses the symptoms of the disease and not the underlying root cause of the disease. Diabetes is reversible, even for insulin-dependent type II diabetics, however most conventional doctors do not know how to reverse the disease process.

If you don't address the root cause or the health issues at a cellular level, then you are not curing the patient, rather you are putting a Band-Aid over the problem. For example, you see your doctor for hypertension. Your mainstream doctor will put you on a blood pressure medication. If you don't take your medication, your blood pressure will rise again. Mainstream physicians don't investigate as to why your blood pressure has gone up. You weren't born with high blood pressure. While you were living your life, something went wrong and your blood pressure, as your body's response (symptom), went up.

Each medication you take has some side effect; some are obvious and some are very subtle. Every medicine depletes your body of certain nutrients. These nutrients are necessary for your cells to function.

After all, your body is made up of trillions of cells, and nutrient deficiencies have a domino effect. As a functional medicine doctor, we look at a health issue at the cellular level. Together, we go back and see what could have happened at a cellular level that led to your high blood pressure.

Could it be your diet?

Are you lacking nutrients?

Is your food contaminated with toxins (pesticides, herbicides)?

Is the soil that your food was grown in depleted of minerals?

Could your gut be sensitive to the food, leading to gut inflammation and poor nutrient absorption?

Could you be taking over-the-counter remedies or prescription medications that interfere with the acid production needed for your nutrient absorption (i.e. Proton Pump Inhibitors)?

Could you have a low-grade infection leading to poor absorption?

Could you have small intestinal bacterial overgrowth (SIBO)?

How about enzyme deficiencies leading to poor absorption? For your foods to be absorbed, you need stomach acid, bile, and enzymes.

In searching for the underlying cause of hypertension we ask:

Could you have oral/dental decay causing a low-grade infection?

Could there be a lack of the appropriate amount and/or type of bacteria in your gastrointestinal tract?

Could there be heavy metals present such as those in dental amalgams?

Could there be a lack of appropriate oils in your cells?

How about low oxygen or energy in your cells?

And of course, let's not forget about your hormones. Could there be an imbalance of your hormones, i.e., cortisol, thyroid, male and female hormones, aldosterone, etc. that led to your hypertension?

AS FUNCTIONAL MEDICINE DOCTORS, WE DIG DEEPER TO RESEARCH THE ROOT CAUSE OF YOUR ILLNESS

Disease care is extremely expensive. In a report in the Boston Globe titled, "Retired Couple May Need $240,000 for Healthcare, the authors calculated what the average out-of-pocket costs for medical expenses would be for a couple who are both 65 years old if they live to their life expectancy; for men, that was 82 years of age, and for women it was 85 years of age. The $240,000 is just the average number, as 50% of those will pay more than $240,000. Living a healthy life style and doing your best to avoid having to use modern medicine very often is one of the best ways to invest in your health, and save money.

Many people take good care of their cars. They service their car and change the damaged auto parts and don't think twice about paying for it. We simply need our vehicles to get around, and it is an investment to take care of our cars. Unfortunately, when it comes to our own health needs, we tend to ignore them and let the insurance companies pay for our illness. Insurance companies pay for illness and not wellness. Isn't it better to prevent major illnesses by being proactive and paying for your own wellness, rather than waiting until a stroke, heart attack, cancer, etc. hits you and then seek medical care? By then, you will most likely have a compromised life with some disabilities.

The wealthiest people in the world will not enjoy their lives if they are ill. Poor health restricts you from enjoying your life, being with people you love, traveling and engaging in your favorite hobbies. I say, "It is worth spending money and staying healthy."

You are worth it!

Chronic diseases will cost the global economy over $47 trillion in the next twenty years. Medicare's unfunded liabilities are estimated at $90 trillion dollars, and Medicare will likely be bankrupt in ten years. The state Medicaid programs are the fastest growing part of state budgets and are going to bankrupt the states. Chronic diseases account for 78% of healthcare spending. We must change our approach to healthcare; functional medicine is the answer to preventing chronic diseases.

The nation as a whole spends almost twice as much on healthcare costs as it does for food. Our food is cheap, easily available, although it is often very poor quality. Approximately 90% of Americans are going to die from a chronic disease that would be preventable by changing their diet and lifestyle. When you look at the cost of food in those terms, you see that our food really is not as cheap as it seems.

There are about a thousand people in the United States who are over 100 years of age. Virtually all of these people have been completely disease-free all of their lives, and they typically have maintained their mental acuity. They also have hormone levels that have stayed at a much higher level than their peers who have died. This is what we should consider as normal. We should all be living long, productive lives and living to 100 should be, and can be, the norm.

I am amazed at how often patients go to other doctors with complaints and the doctor tells them that's normal for their age. If you went to an optometrist and he said your vision is 20/80 and then said well that's normal for your age so I'm not going to give you glasses, would you find that acceptable? Obviously 20/20 vision is normal. It is not normal to have high blood pressure; that is not a normal state for the human body. It is not normal to have depression or high oxidized cholesterol either. Depression is not caused by a Prozac deficiency, nor is high cholesterol caused by a Lipitor deficiency. Both of these conditions are symptoms of some underlying biochemical imbalance. If you correct the imbalance, then the symptoms resolve without using any prescription drugs. Prescription drugs do not cure diseases. They may "cure" a symptom for a day, until you have to take another dose the next day. Imagine if your "check engine" light went on in your car and you took it to the mechanic, and he reset the light; but the next day it was back on. Would you go back to the mechanic every day for him to reset the "check engine" light? Or would you find the root cause of the light going on and fix it instead? Taking a pill every day is equivalent to resetting your "check engine" light every day.

Many times a patient goes to the doctor and describes a symptom: "Doctor, I have pain in all my muscles." The doctor says, "I know what you have. You have fibromyalgia." In case you didn't know, your doctor has just repeated your symptoms back to you in Latin (or Greek.) (fibro is Latin for "fibrous tissue." "Myalgia" is Greek for "muscle pain").

Occasionally patients are given a diagnosis that isn't a real diagnosis. Cryptogenic cirrhosis is an example. Cryptogenic is from the Greek "krypt," or hidden, and "genesis," or origin. Therefore, the diagnosis is unknown. Any diagnosis that begins with "idiopathic" is a non-diagnosis. Idiopathic means "arising from an unknown cause." Don't accept these non-diagnosis from a healthcare provider. There is a root cause.

Stay proactive and seek health advice from a functional medicine provider.

Chapter Two

✎ **STEP 2** ✎

THINK POSITIVE

Your thoughts affect your brain cells and your gene expressions. Research completed in 2013 at UCLA and the University of North Carolina, showed that positive psychology impacts human gene expression. Every time you think positively, your brain releases a peptide from your posterior pituitary gland which travels through your body and heals your cells. Every time you think negatively, your brain releases a different peptide which travels throughout your body and destroys your cells. These peptides also affect your genetic expressions.

Genetic expression needs to be explained. What most of us have been taught about DNA is not really accurate. We were told that our DNA is like a blueprint given to us when we are conceived and we cannot change it. A better explanation is that our DNA is like a library filled with 100,000 sets of blueprints. When a cell needs to make a protein, it goes to the library and pulls out a set of blueprints to make whatever protein it needs to make. The set of blueprints that it pulls out _**can**_ change. That is genetic expression. The two main ways to alter genetic expression are from diet and exercise. A poor diet or lack of exercise will cause bad genes to be expressed. In other words, genes can be switched on and off by changes in your environment. Also, the bad gene expression can be passed down to children and grandchild. Epigenetics is the study of inheritable changes in genetic expression. It is very important that women of child-bearing age live a healthy lifestyle so they do not pass down poor gene-expression to their offspring.

You may have the gene for a health condition but as long as you don't have the environment, you won't express that gene. As the genetic technology has advanced, we now know that genes alone usually are not powerful enough to cause a disease; neither is the environment alone. So generally, we need both pieces of the puzzle to get a specific disease.

Gene + environment = disease

For example, a patient revealed to me that her grandmother smoked two packs of cigarettes for over 70 years and did not get lung cancer and died at age 103. On the other hand, we hear of patients who have never smoked but died of lung cancer. So how do you make sense of this? For an answer, lets revisit the above formula: gene + environment = disease.

In the patient's grandmother's case, she did not have the gene for lung cancer but she had the environment (smoking). In turn, she did not get lung cancer. In the person who never smoked and got lung cancer, he had the gene and his environment included a second-hand smoker situation. As a child, both of his parents smoked, and during his adulthood, his roommates smoked. Although he did not smoke, his environment was a smoker environment and he was a victim of second-hand smoke which led to his lung cancer. I believe genes are over-rated as an explanation for disease.

Your good genes are expressed when you think positively and your bad genes are expressed when you think negatively. Your brain cell receptors will be occupied by these peptides. The more bad peptides you release, the more cell receptors you occupy, leaving less space for good peptides to bind to receptors. This translates into the more negatively you think, the more negative your life becomes and vice versa. It is very hard for you as a pessimistic person to become optimistic since you have to over-produce enough "happy" peptides to occupy more and more receptors, leaving less room for "grumpy" peptides.

The process of learning to think positively can take over three months and you will need special training to help get you there. There are several ways to address this issue of positive thinking such as motivational tapes, seminars, books, etc., along with minimizing your relationships with negative people around you. An experienced therapist can also be very helpful.

15

Another method to learn to think positively is by use of QEEG and neurofeedback training. This is a computerized device where a cap is placed on your head and electrodes from the cap are attached to the computer. The computer then maps your brain and gives the provider information about your brain waves (alpha, beta, delta, and theta) and whether they are in balance with one another in different parts of your brain.

Based on the neuro map results, the computer will create a neuro feedback program for you to balance your brain waves. This involves placing two electrodes on your head that are attached to a computer. You will then wear a pair of glasses that emit light. During this time, you can watch a movie on the computer screen. While you are trying to see the screen, your vision will be fuzzy and your brain has to work to overcome the blurriness so that you can have a clear vision for your movie. This is a very effective device to reverse depression, anxiety, attention deficit disorder, traumatic brain injury, post-traumatic stress disorder, etc.

Neuro feedback can also be used for all of the following problems:

- mood disorders such as major depression and bipolar disorder

- obsessive compulsive disorder (OCD)

- Lyme disease

- tinnitus

- tremor

- pain

- insomnia

- eating disorders and binging

- addictions

- autism

- schizophrenia

- Alzheimer's dementia

- Parkinson's disease and more

Many teachers diagnose young students who are not attentive or cooperative in school as having attention deficit disorder (ADD) and demand that the child's parents take him or her to a psychiatrist so that Ritalin can be started. Ritalin has been overly used in children diagnosed with ADD or ADHD. Some doctors do not investigate the child's behavior before starting amphetamine like drugs, even though the diagnosis requires at least six months of observation before the diagnosis can be made. There are cases of children with a brain tumor, hormonal imbalances, nutrient deficiencies, environmental toxicity, poor home environment, high stress provoking situations, etc. that were placed on amphetamines based on the teacher's or psychiatrist's recommendation. These concerned parents will do anything to help their children, and by trusting the teacher or the psychiatrist without a full medical and psychological workup, their children can be misdiagnosed and mistreated.

One of my patients, Lauren, was telling me that her son's eighth grade teacher had threatened her and her husband that their son would not advance to ninth grade unless he was started on Ritalin. She told me her son is extremely bright and is easily bored if not challenged. Lauren had discussed this with her son's private school's teachers, principal and school psychologist and had requested that her son be given more advanced educational tasks so that he could be challenged, which in turn would help him not distract others in the classroom. Her pleas were ignored and she was never given another option. Lauren and her husband researched the causes of hyperactivity and found a psychologist who utilized computerized testing to diagnose learning behaviors. After many visits to the psychologist, her son was diagnosed with a very high IQ and recommended to be placed in a more challenging environment.

This brings us back to whether you are going to trust your teacher to misdiagnose your child and place him or her on a heavy-duty stimulant with lots of adverse effects. In the case of my patient Lauren, she had the time and the money to take the matter into her own hands and not follow the teacher's recommendations. She also told me that while her son was being evaluated, she learned about nonpharmacological treatment options for children with ADD/ADHD which includes brain-mapping (QEEG) and neurofeedback.

Another very important intensive treatment for ADD/ADHD children is to improve their diet. Getting children off sugars, grains, dairy, and bad fats such as trans-fats and vegetable oils has helped these children to be able to focus and function in a healthy manner. These powerful nonprescription options are not typically discussed by teachers or doctors to help these children and their families.

Another diagnosis modality is a brain SPECT imaging (single photon emission computed tomography) which looks at blood flow to the brain and identifies any over-or under-active regions of the brain. A brain SPECT not only can help with the diagnosis, but also can help in guiding the treatment. This is extremely useful for the diagnosis of traumatic brain injury (TBI), also known as concussions, which is the leading cause of death or disability in the population under 45-years of age. A Brain SPECT is more sensitive than a brain MRI or CT scan for traumatic brain injury patients. You can find further information on SPECT scan at Dr. Amen's clinics nationwide. Therefore, putting the patient on antidepressant or antianxiety medications without further workup or options can lead to many serious health problems.

Another tool is a functional MRI (fMFI) which shows what part of the brain is active in response to the patient's task performance. FMRI is used in autism, pre-and post-neurosurgery procedures, Alzheimer's disease, schizophrenia, OCD, ADD/ADHD and major depressive disorders.

Meditation, singing, exercising, laughter, cuddling and touching, deep breathing, owning a loving pet, being around positive people and listening to motivational tapes or seminars can all increase your brain's good peptides.

In summary, neural plasticity can change the structure and function of your brain. **Repetitive positive thoughts and activities can rewire your brain and strengthen brain areas that stimulate positive feelings.** We have the power to achieve anything if we stop negative thoughts and focus on positive thoughts. You should avoid negative words such as "can't", "won't", "impossible", and instead use positive words such as "I can", "I will" and "if there is a will, there is a way". Try to avoid worrying, as overthinking about a problem causes anxiety which lasts for days and drains your energy and affects your health in many negative ways. The more you focus on problems the more you strengthen the negative peptide release. Make a goal for yourself to stop thinking negatively now and build it up a little at a time every day. Over time, your brain will become more positive which will not only affect you, but will also affect your environment and you will notice good things start to happen to you.

Your thoughts affect your physiology. You need to be positive and focus on things to be grateful for. Chronic negative thoughts harm your health. **Use positive affirmations every day.** Seek natural methods for brain health, such as using amino acids, and B vitamins, particularly vitamins B6, folate, and B12. Many times, the root cause of brain dysfunction originates in the GI tract, or is caused from some immune system dysfunction.

Chapter Three

❧ **STEP 3** ❧

BALANCING YOUR HORMONES

There is an ideal hormonal blueprint for everyone and it's not one-size-fits-all.

What are hormones? Hormones are chemicals that we produce in our glands and cells that are released into the bloodstream, which in turn regulate specific organs. Hormones are messengers that control the cell's functions. They are extremely powerful and a very small amount can have major physiologic and psychologic effects.

A mainstream physician will tell you that as you age, your hormones decline. A functional medicine doctor will tell you that you age *because* your hormones decline. Every physical sign of aging is a hormone deficiency. Every wrinkle, loose skin, grey hair, etc., is a sign of a hormone deficiency.

For you to avoid dying prematurely, you need to look and feel younger and have a firm body. Bioidentical hormone therapy is one of the cornerstones to make that happen.

The Chinese started using bioidentical hormones over 3,000 years ago. They collected urine from healthy teenage boys and girls, dried, purified and mixed it with dates to form pills. If that sounds disgusting, you should be aware that Premarin, a common synthetic hormone given to post-menopausal women, is extracted from horse urine. In fact that is where it gets its name; it stands for PREgnant MARes uRINe.

While exact numbers are unknown, it is estimated there are between 20,000-50,000 mares world-wide that are kept pregnant, and their urine is collected to make Premarin and PremPro. Estrogens from horses are not the same as those in humans, and although they have a similar effect on estrogen receptors, the human body cannot eliminate them properly. Synthetic hormones can therefore cause long-term health risks, as the Women's Health Initiative (WHI) showed almost 20 years ago. This was a study done from 1993 – 1998 with over 161,000 post-menopausal women using Premarin and Prempro, which is a synthetic estrogen and progesterone hormone derived from horse urine. This study was originally designed to be a 10-year study, but due to the significant increase in strokes, part of the study was stopped; they mistakenly blamed estrogen as the problem. However, part of the study continued and the results of that data showed progestin, which is the synthetic form of progesterone, to be the culprit for this disaster. Despite the complications, this drug was never taken off the market and is still available today by prescription.

Bio-identical hormones are actually manufactured from yams and altered such that the molecules are identical to what the human body produces. In other words, they are quite safe and we don't have to collect the urine from a bunch of teenagers to obtain them. The fear of breast cancer is unfounded from bio-identical hormones. Estrogens do not cause cancer. If they did, you'd see young women in their teens and 20's with breast cancer when their estrogens are at the highest level. The link between hormones and cancer appears to be from problems with poor estrogen metabolism and elimination. It is the byproduct from the breakdown of estrogens that appears to increase the risk and not from the hormones themselves. You should have your hormones monitored via urine tests to measure the metabolites.

Keeping your hormones at youthful levels, either through lifestyle changes and/or by the use of bio-identical hormone replacement therapy, is the foundation for longevity.

Your hormones are like a symphony. If they are all working well together, your music will sound great, but if one of the instruments is off tune, your music will sound unpleasant and that is exactly how you will feel inside. I am not just talking about your estrogen, progesterone, or testosterone. I mean all of your hormones, including your thyroid, adrenal, pancreatic, ovarian, testicular, pineal, pituitary, etc.

Some of your major hormones are derived from cholesterol, such as pregnenolone, progesterone, testosterone, DHEA, aldosterone, cortisol, and estrogens. Each of these hormones play a great role in your health and vitality.

Pregnenolone and progesterone help with your brain function, to improve memory, sleep, and anxiety.

DHEA is sometimes called the "fountain of youth" hormone. It is an anabolic hormone (builds the cells) and has many favored actions. Testosterone is known to be a male hormone but it is also present in females and works in muscle building, memory, respiration, bone building, heart function, libido, erection, ejaculation, and male sexual characters.

Aldosterone is a water and salt balancing hormone. You cannot live without it and it also affects your blood pressure.

Estrogens are major female hormones. They play a big role in memory and bone building, but affect every organ. A common myth conveyed by conventional physicians is that hormones cause heart attacks, strokes, and breast cancer. This may be true with synthetic hormones, but it's completely false when it comes to bio-identical hormones. Keep in mind that the highest amount of female or male hormones are seen in the young at puberty. How many 14- to 16-year-olds do you know that have had heart attacks, strokes, breast or prostate cancer? Our hormone levels decline during the aging process.

In the postmenopausal female, estrogen equals memory. In the post-andropausal male, testosterone equals memory. Keeping your hormones at youthful levels is required to keep your memory intact as you age.

There are two leading health conditions that will take your independence away and lead you to a nursing home. The first is a hip or pelvic fracture usually due to osteoporosis (severe bone loss). The second is Alzheimer's disease. Both of these conditions could be prevented if the patient's physicians addressed these health issues before they ever occurred. A low-fat diet or taking statin medications for cholesterol leading to low cholesterol levels, especially under 140 mg/dL, will decrease the production of hormones that are needed for the brain to keep your memory intact and your bones to stay strong enough to prevent osteoporosis.

The most important time for a women to be on bio-identical hormone therapy is immediately before and after menopause. Half of a women's total bone loss in life occurs in the first two years after menopause. Hormone therapy should not be delayed because hormone receptors start to diminish from non-use, so starting bio-identical hormone replacement many years after menopause is not as effective as starting at menopause.

Another endocrine organ is the pancreas. Your pancreas produces insulin, amylin and glucagon. These hormones play a major role in blood and cellular sugar levels.

Excess sugar is very toxic to every organ in our body. Many people think sugar is only in cookies, ice cream, chocolate or candy. Many of my patients are surprised to find out that fruits are mostly sugar. Wine is another routinely consumed beverage that increases your blood sugar. Grains, such as bread, pasta, and rice, convert into sugar in your body. When you consume sugar, insulin is released from your pancreas and stores the sugar inside of cells. We then utilize the stored sugar for energy. Insulin signals fat cells to absorb fat that is circulating in the blood. Basically, it makes your fat cells become fatter. Insulin also tells the liver to convert glucose into fat. Eating excess sugar leads to insulin resistance. This in turn leads to many maladies associated with metabolic syndrome. Excess sugar in the blood travels through your body, harming many organs such as eyes, kidneys, liver, blood vessels, brain, etc. This is why a poorly controlled diabetic person can become blind, suffer amputated limbs, be on dialysis with kidney failure, or suffer from an early heart attack or stroke. Diabetic patients also suffer from a liver abnormality called fatty liver which can advance to liver cirrhosis. There is going to be an epidemic of liver failure from excessive sugar consumption. Fructose is a leading cause of fatty liver and the obesity epidemic.

The new name for Alzheimer's disease is diabetes type III. Excess sugar travels in your blood vessels and crosses the blood-brain barrier. Excessive sugar harms brain cells. Over the years, you will lose enough brain cells so that when you walk into your home, you might look at your family and say "Who are you people." This is called Alzheimer's disease.

Did you know that by controlling your blood sugar you can partially or completely reverse these conditions? There are also some intravenous therapies that can reverse damage to these organs: vitamin C, Alpha-lipoic acid, phosphatidyl-choline, B vitamins and major auto hemotherapy (MAH). These IV therapies have been shown to aid in the healing process of these organs affected by high blood sugar. Your functional medicine provider can guide you to find these nonconventional therapies that are not sought after or mentioned by a conventional physician. It is not because your doctor is hiding this information from you, rather they are unaware of these options existing. Mainstream physicians tend to not recommend these ideal treatment options because they are unfamiliar with the treatments and are concerned about the possibility of harm to their patients.

I know many conventional physicians who have tried to get my patients off successful nonconventional therapies since they are not knowledgeable in the field of functional medicine. Some conventional doctors when asked about a nonconventional therapy, talk the patient out of the treatment by convincing the patient they will be harmed by such therapies. Very few conventional physicians tell their patients, "I am not familiar with that treatment, but I would love to learn about it and give you my opinion." Interestingly enough, this is how I became aware of functional medicine. When practicing conventional medicine, my patients would ask me about nonconventional therapies of which I was unaware and unfamiliar with their existence. Therefore, I would tell my patients, "I don't know enough to give you an accurate response. Let me research it." While doing such research, *a whole new world of medicine opened up to me.*

Another major gland is your pituitary gland. This is a pea-sized gland at the base of your brain; it produces many different hormones, including the following and their role in our health:

- Growth hormone: this hormone promotes growth by stimulating cells to grow and divide, increasing muscle and bone growth as well as protein synthesis.

- Prolactin: this hormone stimulates milk production for breast-feeding women and has an action on the reproductive and the immune system.

- Follicular stimulating hormone (FSH): this hormone regulates the release of eggs from the ovaries in women, and the testosterone and sperm production in men, and has an action on the immune system.

- Luteinizing Hormone (LH): it regulates the female menstrual cycle and works with FSH to produce sperm in men.

- Adrenocorticotrophic hormone (ACTH): this hormone regulates cortisol levels released from the adrenal gland which is a key factor in the body's metabolism of fats, carbohydrates, sodium and potassium, protein, and blood pressure.

- Thyroid stimulating hormone (TSH): this hormone causes the thyroid gland to make the thyroid hormones T3 and T4 which control our body's metabolism.

The above six hormones are produced from the anterior pituitary gland.

The posterior pituitary gland produces the following two hormones:

- Oxytocin: this hormone is also known as the love hormone or cuddle hormone and is needed for de-stressing. Oxytocin helps people socially and promotes the mother-child bonding. Even playing with your pet will increase your oxytocin levels. This hormone affects your emotions, cognition, and social behaviors. Oxytocin is also used in lactation and uterine contraction during childbirth. One of the most important roles for oxytocin is with the production of nitric oxide, which protects your blood vessels from plaque formation in arteries (atherosclerosis.)

- Antidiuretic hormone (ADH): this hormone has an antidiuretic action that prevents the production of dilute urine and maintains blood pressure, blood volume and the tissue's water content.

An excess or deficiency of any of these hormones can cause different medical conditions which require treatment.

Cortisol is the major stress hormone and as with the other hormones, either an excess or deficiency of this hormone can lead to major health issues. It is the most potent hormone in the body. It is also the most abundant hormone in the body. Chronic elevation of cortisol is one of the most destructive forces in our body. It causes aging and wear and tear, and can cause insulin resistance. Every chronic illness is either caused by stress, or exacerbated by chronic stress.

Melatonin is one of the most interesting and effective antiaging hormones. Melatonin has been found in a species of bacteria that dates back 2-3.5 billion years, making melatonin one of the oldest biochemical molecules on earth. It is found in every living plant and animal species on earth. It has independent functions in the body separate from its role as a hormone, such as its antioxidant properties. Therefore, melatonin should be classified as both a vitamin and a hormone.

Most people are aware of the role of melatonin with sleep. It is mainly produced in the brain, stored in a pineal gland and released throughout the night. It helps you fall asleep and stay asleep. But melatonin has many other roles in the body, and we always have melatonin in our system. It is one of the most potent immune modulators in the human body. In high doses it can both treat and prevent cancer.

Melatonin is the only hormone that you can take that does not appear to suppress your body's normal production of the hormone. There are no known serious complications from it. There is no known LD50 for melatonin. LD50 is how researchers establish toxicity for a substance. It determines what the lethal dose is for 50% of the subjects. In animal studies, they have given the equivalent of 80,000 mg to a 220 lb. subject, with no problems. Melatonin may be the only substance known that has no LD50.

What are the health benefits of melatonin? Melatonin is a powerful antioxidant. It has neuroprotective effects and is a potent immune modulator. It decreases viral infections and arterial plaque formation (atherosclerosis) and it has anticancer attributes. It is also a mitochondrial resuscitator, which gives you more energy at the cellular level. In children, it has been used to treat mood disorders as well as help those with learning disabilities. It is helpful in the treatment of macular degeneration, dementia, Parkinson's, atherosclerosis and cancer.

Melatonin is a hormone sensitizer and there is evidence that it may be a decline in melatonin levels that trigger menopause and other hormone deficiencies. Indeed, one study showed that menopause could actually be reversed by taking melatonin. One study with melatonin supplementation of women ages 42 to 62 showed increased thyroid hormone levels and suppressed Luteinizing Hormone (LH) levels. Subjects in the study reported a general improvement in mood and a significant reduction of depression. Restoration of pituitary and thyroid functions were also noted.

Melatonin easily crosses all cell membranes, including the mitochondrial cell membrane and the blood-brain barrier. It stimulates energy production in your mitochondria, which power every cell in our body.

Melatonin has been found to prevent neuronal death caused by exposure to the amyloid beta protein, which is present in Alzheimer's disease. This suggests that melatonin might prevent Alzheimer's.

Inflammation is one of the causes of early aging. Melatonin decreases age-related inflammatory cells to youthful levels.

Melatonin is an anticancer hormone. It inhibits cancer cell growth in <u>vitro</u> in multiple human cancers, and it prevents carcinogen-induced DNA damage rendering them safe. Melatonin doses for cancer treatment are kept at high levels throughout the day.

Contrary to common belief, melatonin does not induce sleep nor make you sleepy by itself. Melatonin stimulates sensitivity to the dark so you must have a dark bedroom to get a good night's sleep. You can take melatonin during the day and it will not make you sleepy.

Melatonin is also effective for restoring normal circadian rhythm and we use it extensively with weight-loss patients. It can also be quite effective for treating migraine headaches.

Melatonin complications, though rare, include restless sleep, insomnia, wild dreams, and grogginess in the morning. Morning grogginess typically only lasts for a few days after starting with a high-dose regimen. You should only use very pure melatonin when using it at high doses. Side effects from melatonin are mostly caused by contaminants in the capsules.

Melatonin is a very important antiaging hormone that is overlooked even by most functional medicine physicians.

Thyroid hormone plays a critical role in aging and longevity. Aging can best be described as a reduction in cellular energy; thyroid is the hormone that drives cellular metabolism. Every cell in your body that has a cell nucleus, requires thyroid hormone. That means every cell in your body, except red and white blood cells, requires thyroid hormone. It drives every single metabolic process in the body. It also regulates your body's temperature. If your body temperature is one degree below normal, you are slowing down every enzymatic process in the body. Of all the bio-markers in the body, the one bio-marker that has the narrowest "normal" range is body temperature. **Many illnesses are merely the manifestations of low thyroid function.**

You cannot be optimally well unless your thyroid is functioning optimally, yet you cannot determine that from a standard thyroid lab test. There are multiple reasons why this is true. Before lab tests were available, doctor's used other methods to determine if the thyroid was low; one such test was body temperature and reflex rate. Once the TSH test was available, the amount of thyroid hormone prescribed by doctors dropped by half because of their reliance on the TSH lab results. Many people who require thyroid hormones are not getting them because their TSH lab tests fall in the "normal" range. It is estimated that about 40% of Americans have sub-optimal thyroid hormone levels, yet only 5% of Americans have thyroid levels that are outside of the current lab ranges.

Body temperature is a great way to determine if your thyroid is sub-optimal. People know that when your body temperature is above normal, something is wrong. Yet doctors routinely ignore anybody with a body temperature that is below normal. **Low body temperature is a very strong indicator of low thyroid function, and it is not normal.**

I often have to explain to patients how labs determine the "normal ranges" indicated on lab reports. What labs do is to take the last 100,000 test results and take two standard deviations above and below the mean of those test results.

34

This means in order to be considered "high," you need to have a value in the top 2.5%, and to be "low" you need to be in the bottom 2.5%. So by definition, 95% of everyone tested on any given lab test **_must be_** in the normal range. Are 95% of Americans healthy? Not even close! In my office we do not rely on lab ranges only. We use the patient's symptoms and their physical findings to help us with the correct diagnosis and proper treatment.

What are the symptoms of low thyroid?

Since thyroid hormone affects every cell in our body, low thyroid levels are associated with many different symptoms. Some of these symptoms or signs include:

- Fatigue
- Weight gain or inability to lose weight
- Depression or anxiety without known cause
- Dizzy spells
- Increased sensitivity to cold
- Constipation and bloating
- Puffy eyes and puffy face
- Course hair/thin hair/hair loss
- Tinnitus (ringing in the ear)
- Memory impairment
- Large tongue

- Goiter or swollen neck
- Premature loss of menstrual cycle in women
- Infertility
- Hoarse voice
- Muscle and joint pain
- Muscle weakness
- Dry skin
- Carpal tunnel
- Thinning of the outer one third of eyebrows
- Swelling in hands and feet
- Paresthesia (numbness and tingling in hands and feet)
- Slow heart rate
- Elevated cholesterol levels
- Delayed puberty
- Poor growth causing short stature
- Poor IQ or mental retardation and birth defect in newborns with mothers suffering from hypothyroidism during pregnancy
- Myxedema which is a life- threatening condition due to long standing undiagnosed hypothyroidism leading to profound lethargy and unconsciousness
- Heart problems such as enlarged heart or heart failure

As you can see by now, low thyroid can have many ill effects and thus needs to be diagnosed and treated. In my clinic, I assess every single patient for low thyroid, and work with them to optimize their thyroid levels.

You may ask what causes low thyroid.

Some of the common causes include medications such as amiodarone (used in irregular heart conditions), lithium (used in psychiatric conditions such as manic disorder), medications used to treat hyperthyroidism (excess thyroid levels), Pituitary gland problems, radiation therapy to the neck, thyroid surgery, auto immune thyroid disease also known as Hashimoto's thyroiditis, viral or bacterial infections affecting thyroid, low iodine, low tyrosine, low progesterone, low selenium, excessive cortisol, chronic infections, and many more.

Most mainstream physicians do not check your hormones and if they do, they only check hormones from one or two organs which are not enough to help find your fountain of youth.

Ask your functional medicine provider to check your hormone levels to make sure your melatonin, growth hormone, insulin, cortisol, progesterone, pregnenolone, and thyroid levels are in the normal range. You may also want to have your provider check for nutrient balance.

Chapter Four

❦ STEP 4 ❧

BIOTRANSFORMATION (DETOXIFICATION)

Medical textbooks discuss biotransformation in great detail. Biotransformation means alteration of chemicals in the body such as medications, toxins, amino acids and nutrients. But the term is rarely used outside of medical school. People instead seem to prefer using the word detoxification. Detoxification is what our body does to neutralize and transform unwanted materials or toxins. We need enzymes, vitamins, minerals, amino acids, healthy gut bacteria, and water for the detoxification systems to work properly.

On a daily basis we are exposed to many toxins in our environment. Our own cells even produce waste products that need to be detoxified and eliminated. We don't always have control over our environment, but we have control over our body's reaction to the toxins in our environment. One of the primary reasons for weight gain is because we cannot detoxify and eliminate substances from our body. When we get exposed to fat-soluble toxic chemicals, our body's response is to protect us by eliminating it if possible, or storing it in a fat cell and then makes us gain fat. If the toxin is water-soluble and cannot be eliminated, our body instead stores the toxin in the extra-cellular matrix (space outside of cells) and causes us to retain water to dilute the toxins. **Therefore, the body's solution to pollution is dilution.** Most overweight or obese people are toxic and thus won't be able to lose or maintain their weight loss until they rid the toxins harbored in their bodies. There are some substances that are called obesogens. Obesogens are substances that make us obese. Some known obesogens include Perfluorooctanoic acid (PFOA) from non-stick cooking surfaces, phthalates, pesticides, herbicides, Bisphenol A (BPA), and Polychlorinated Biphenyls (PCBs).

If you were to Google "obesity by county" and look at the images, you would see some very interesting maps. It shows high rates of obesity in the Great Plains region, and the rates increase the closer the county is to the mouth of the Mississippi river. The herbicide glyphosate (Roundup) is used extensively in the Great Plains, and washes into the Mississippi river, and municipal water treatment do not remove it. Up to 700 parts per billion are allowed in municipal water. Studies with rats show harmful effects at levels 17,000 lower than the allowed limited in drinking water.

The environmental toxins vary from foods that have been contaminated with food coloring or additives, pesticides and herbicides, mold, heavy metals (mercury in dental amalgams or in the contaminated seafood), plastic containers, paper coating, air pollutants, lotions, creams, topical makeup, hair dyes, hair sprays, shampoos/conditioners, hair products, eyelash extension glues or dyes, permanent makeup dye, fluoride in toothpaste, soaps, candles, nail polish, laundry fabric softeners, Scotch Gard/fabric and carpet protectors, flame retardant in furniture or electronics, wood preservatives, DDT (which has been banned but has continued to persist in our environment for decades), and much more.

A large-scale international study of 43,000 men showed that in the period 1973-2011, sperm rates dropped by 50-60%, and have continued to decline. Low sperm-rates are linked to all-cause mortality, and it is believed that endocrine disruptors and pesticides are the likely cause of the decline. Endocrine disruptors are substances that act like hormones in the body, such as BPA from plastics, and the herbicide glyphosate (Roundup).

Twenty-five percent of teenage girls suffer from urinary incontinence due to imbalance of their hormones from environmental endocrine disruptors.

Studies have shown newborn umbilical cord blood is contaminated with 287 toxic chemicals, 180 of which are shown to cause cancer, 217 of which are toxic to the central nervous system and brain, and 208 of which are the toxins associated with birth defects. Some of these chemicals mimic our own hormones and cause hormonal disruption leading to sterility and/or infertility.

One of my patient's three-month old daughter was diagnosed with a very aggressive cancer that usually affects young men. Upon investigation, it was determined that the baby contracted the cancer *in utero*.

As you can see, we live in an environment that is quite toxic. We are even exposed to these toxins before we are born. It is our responsibility to detoxify these chemicals out of our bodies on a regular basis in order for us to stay healthy.

We have five organs that detoxify us on a daily basis. As long as these organs function properly, we should be able to get rid of most toxic materials. I am not talking about someone pouring cyanide in your drink and overloading your toxic system, rather your day-to-day toxic exposures.

The most-important organ involved in detoxifying our body is our **liver**. The liver acts like a factory, altering toxins to either enter back into our blood for kidneys to filter them, or excreted into the bowel to be eliminated in the feces. However, in the case of fat soluble compounds, your liver will break it down differently using certain nutrients. Methylation is a basic process in the body. It is how our body passes a water-soluble substance through a fat-soluble membrane, such as a cell membrane, or a nerve sheath, or a mitochondrial membrane. The methylation process adds a methyl donor to a molecule. There are over 250 methylation cycles in the human body, including getting energy in and out of mitochondria, DNA replication, making neurotransmitters, and detoxifying estrogens.

Vitamin B12 and folate play a major role in every methylation pathway. Many of us have genetic mutations that may affect our methylation. These mutations can affect our detoxification of fat soluble compounds via the liver. These mutations can be detected by genetic testing, such as 23andMe.com. You can obtain the kit online without prescription or order from your physician. Once the test is done, which is easily completed by a swab sample from your mouth, you need to pay a different lab to translate the genetic mutations into a sensible language for you. There are many genetic companies that are available online, and the fees are reasonable.

The second-most organ that protects us against toxins is our **gut**. We eat different foods which get absorbed in different parts of our gastrointestinal tract. We need stomach acid, pancreatic enzymes, bile, amylase, and lipase to absorb our foods. The microbiome, which are the friendly bacteria in our gut, are extremely helpful in digesting and absorbing our nutrients. Due to the overuse of antibiotics and the lack of fiber in our diet, we often lack appropriate gut bacteria. A healthy gut will contain one hundred trillion bacteria. There must be the right balance of bacteria for our gut to remain healthy. These bacteria influence every system in our body in a positive manner. They help with digestion by decreasing gas and bloating, and help us absorb nutrients. They improve our immune system, make vitamins, and transform food into energy. They help us detoxify, lower our bad cholesterol, prevent osteoporosis, help us lose weight, and much more. Our gut will excrete the toxins so that they are eliminated via feces. It is normal to have one bowel movement per meal. If you eat breakfast, lunch, and dinner you should have three bowel movements a day. If you have any less than that, you are likely holding onto toxins. Another problem is slow bowel transit time. Normal bowel transit time takes about 18 hours from eating to elimination. A simple test is to eat some beets and see how long it take to show up in your stool. If it takes more than 24 hours, you have slow transit time, and are more likely to reabsorb toxins.

I have had patients who were having one bowel movement a week. These patients were extremely toxic. If you don't eliminate your toxic ingested foods, your body will reabsorb the toxins from your intestines into your blood stream and make you more toxic. There are many causes why one may not eliminate as often as needed. Some examples are food sensitivities such as gluten and dairy, hormonal imbalances such as hypoactive thyroid, sedentary lifestyle, medications, lack of certain nutrients such as magnesium, inappropriate number and/or type of microbiome, stress and emotional conditions, dehydration, intestinal infections, especially with candida (which is a type of fungus) and much more.

It is important to avoid eating the foods that may be causing gut inflammation, leading to inability to expel the toxins or absorb nutrients. I recommend that my patients get intravenous nutritional therapies while they are working on healing their gut. Do your best to eat organic, non-GMO foods as much as possible. There are multiple tests available to check for food sensitivities. It is also important to take prebiotics (fiber) and probiotics on daily basis (greater than 30 billion). I also advise my patients to change their probiotics every three months so that they can populate their gut with different types of bacteria since each microbiome has different functions. If my patients are placed on antibiotics, I encourage them to increase their probiotic intake. Rectal ozone insufflation is also extremely helpful in detoxifying through the GI tract. This is an excellent way to keep the liver functioning well. Another very important way to detoxify, is colonics. I recommend you seek a licensed colonic therapist who can customize your colonics based on your health history.

Since we house 70% of our immune system and 90% of our serotonin receptors in our gut, we need to take good care of our gastrointestinal tract. **Good health begins in the GUT.**

The third organ responsible for detoxification is our **skin**. We detoxify by sweating and expelling toxins through our skin pores. Exercising, leading to sweating, helps to get rid of some of the toxins. However, we don't exercise or sweat enough to overcome our environmental toxins. Far-infrared sauna is helpful in making us sweat more. Spending an hour in a far-infrared sauna at least three times a week has been proven to decrease the toxic load in our body. Ironically, some far-infrared saunas are made of certain wood or wood preservatives and glues that are more toxic to our system. Therefore, if you plan to buy a far-infrared sauna, you need to do your research and look for one that is made of non-toxic materials.

Far-infrared saunas heat your body from inside out and make you sweat a great deal. You can adjust the temperature starting lower and slowly increasing the temperature as tolerated. Most people tolerate this heat well since it's a dry heat, and the air does not heat up as much as your body. Of course, it is recommended that you hydrate with mineral water prior and after your sauna. You must be able to shower immediately after you are done. There are some facilities that offer Far-infrared sauna but do not have showers available in their facility.

Ozone sauna is another type of sauna that can help detoxify many environmental toxins; we recommend 30 – 60 minutes twice a week for 14 weeks. It is best to receive intravenous fluids with vitamins and minerals immediately after the sauna. If that option is not available to you, then try to hydrate with mineral water before and after using the sauna.

The fourth set of organs that help us detoxify, are our **lungs**. Imagine you're going to an event and you want to wear that beautiful red dress. On the day of the event you realize that your dress is at the dry cleaners and you are short on time. You decide to stop by the dry cleaners and pick up your dress and change in their bathroom. Once you do that, you will absorb the solvents and other toxins through your skin into your body. Your lungs will try to protect you by shifting the solvents out of your body through exhaling.

The fifth set of organs that protect us against toxins are our **kidneys**. Every drop of blood gets filtered through our kidneys. Our kidneys filter out water-soluble toxins and make urine. Every time you urinate, you are getting rid of some toxins. It is recommended that you drink mineral water to hydrate so that your kidneys will function optimally. In normal, functioning kidneys, we recommend you drink half your body weight in ounces per day. For example, if you weigh 140 pounds, you should be drinking 70 ounces of mineral water per day. To get mineral water, you can add a pinch of sea salt to each 8-ounce glass containing filtered water. It is not recommended that you add refined salt or table salt to your water or your foods. Do not use plastic cups and avoid unfiltered water.

Chapter Five

❧ **STEP 5** ❧

LIFE STYLE CHANGES

DIET

Diet and exercise must be modified to increase longevity. This concept is not one-size-fits-all, but needs to be individualized. For instance, telling a patient to drink a lot of water can be fatal if the patient suffers from congestive heart failure or from an obsessive-compulsive disorder and drinks obsessive amounts of water.

Refined salt (table salt) in high amounts is harmful to your body, but sea salt is good for you since it contains a lot of minerals. The "dirtier" the salt, the more minerals it contains and the more health benefits you will have. I would advise changing your household salt to sea salt or some type of mineral salt like Celtic sea salt or Himalayan salt. Observational studies show that you live longer if you consume 4-6 grams of salt a day. A recent study showed that some people have hypertension because they lack sodium, but most doctors tell patients with hypertension to lower their sodium intake. The sodium/potassium ratio is more important than total sodium intake.

Eating trans-fats is very harmful to you. I generally do not recommend a low-fat diet, because low-fat means a high carbohydrate diet. The low-fat diet was introduced in 1976 by our government. In one study, completed by a scientist named Ancel Keys Ph.D., it showed a correlation of saturated fat intake and cardiovascular disease from six countries. However, Dr. Keys had data from 22 countries but the study didn't include results from all 22 countries. If it had, it would have shown that there was a weak correlation between saturated fat consumption and cardiovascular disease. Indeed, there have been numerous human clinical trials on saturated fat and cardiovascular disease and none of them have shown a link. There was also a known link between sugar intake and cardiovascular disease, but the sugar industry was paying for Ancel Keys' research at the time. In 2016, historical analysis of internal industry documents from the sugar industry going back to the 1960's show they influenced researchers to blame heart disease on fat instead of on sugar, including Ancel Keyes.

Based on bad data from Dr. Keys' study, the US government recommended a low-fat diet and lowering dietary cholesterol intake. Since then, obesity and diabetes have been on a sharp incline. What we know now that we did not know then, is that fat does not make you fat. Also, fat does not increase bad cholesterol. Dietary saturated fat often lowers cholesterol levels. I had one patient with a cholesterol level of 356. She could not tolerate statins and other cholesterol lowering medications. I put her on a high saturated fat diet. Her cholesterol dropped to 180 after four months of the high fat diet. Cholesterol has been unfairly demonized. In 2015 the US government removed the dietary restriction on cholesterol. Eating cholesterol doesn't raise cholesterol levels in the blood for most people.

Sugar is the real culprit for cardiovascular disease, not saturated fat. This has been known by some doctors for over 50 years. Sucrose is table sugar and it is comprised of one molecule of glucose and one molecule of fructose. Interestingly, nobody had bothered to do a study to determine if it was the glucose or the fructose that was the problem. A study was finally done recently, and it found that fructose is the molecule that causes most of the metabolic damage to our body. Fructose can only be metabolized by the liver. No other tissue can use it. In high amounts, fructose is toxic to the liver. Fructose is converted into glucose and fatty acids by the liver. It causes fatty liver disease. Fatty liver progresses to nonalcoholic steatohepatitis (NASH). NASH progresses to liver cirrhosis and then liver failure and death.

Patients are being placed on cholesterol lowering medications, such as statins, that have major side effects. Statins deplete your cells of their fuel. For example, if your car does not have any fuel, it won't run. Likewise, your cells do not function properly if your mitochondria does not have enough CoQ10, their "fuel."

Statins (Lipitor, Crestor, Zocor, Pravachol, etc.) will deplete your mitochondria of its CoQ10. If you must be on statins, you must supplement with CoQ10 (at least 300 mg per day). Over and over again, I see patients with severe illnesses that stem from taking cholesterol medications.

Cholesterol is the mother of so many of our essential hormones. When you decrease your total cholesterol to less than 140, your body will have problems making certain hormones that are necessary for your fountain of youth. Cholesterol levels tend to rise as you age because your body is trying to make more hormones because hormones are declining. When I start patients on hormone replacement therapy, their total cholesterol tends to drop.

Your liver makes about 70% of your cholesterol and your diet provides the other 30%. The more cholesterol you eat, the less your liver has to make. Some of your major hormones are derived from cholesterol such as pregnenolone, DHEA, testosterone, aldosterone, cortisol, and estrogens.

While testosterone is known as a male hormone, it is also present in females; it works in muscle building, memory, respiration, bone building, libido, erection, ejaculation, male sexual characters, etc.

Let's talk about my patient Mr. Dave White. Dave is a 56-year-old gentleman with a history of type II diabetes and coronary artery disease. He had a coronary stent in one of his heart arteries two years ago. I see Dave at least every three months and we discuss his diet and blood sugar levels. During my last visit with Dave, I asked him for his food journal and blood sugar levels. He said, "Dr. Shaban, I don't have them today." I asked, "Why not?" He responded, "My blood sugar device is upstairs." I said "So"!!! Dave responded, "I haven't been able to climb up my stairs." I said, "What? How long has that been going on?" Dave said, "It has been two months." I responded, "Oh my goodness, did you call my office to let me know?" He said, "I wanted to, but I thought it would go away eventually." I asked, "Did it?" Dave responded "No. After one month I realized it hadn't gone away and I was going to call you, but I realized I had this appointment coming up in one month. So, I waited."

I decided not to ruminate over his delay in informing me, therefore I said, "Let's go back three months and tell me what had changed."

"Did you start a new job?"

"Did you start on a new medication or supplements?"

"Did you move into a new house?"

"Did you clean your carpets?"

"Did you paint your walls?"

"Have you been working with any toxins such as paint?"

"Have you been traveling?"

"Have you had any recent infections such as flu or gastrointestinal discomforts?"

"Have you tried any new food or delicacies?"

The answer to all of my questions was" No".

He did, however, remember seeing his cardiologist who ran some blood work on him and noticed his total cholesterol and his bad cholesterol were mildly elevated. So, his cardiologist, Dr. Brown, increased Dave's Lipitor (cholesterol medication) from 10 mg a day to 80 mg a day.

"Aha….. I know exactly what has happened. With the increase in your Lipitor dose, your cholesterol has dropped so low that your body cannot make sufficient amounts of testosterone. Since testosterone is needed for muscle strength and movement, you are having a hard time climbing the stairs." I immediately checked his cholesterol and testosterone levels and sure enough, his cholesterol was 50 (lab range is less than 200), but levels under 140 will cause hormonal problems. Dave's testosterone level was barely detectable.

I went over the steroidogenic pathway chart which shows biochemical pathways at a cellular level. I told him since his cholesterol was so low, his body wasn't making enough testosterone to help him with his muscle strength. It also explains Dave's "flat affect" as testosterone is needed for feeling joyous and having a sharp memory.

I reassured him that his condition could be reversed since the change in his medication dose was fairly recent. I then called his cardiologist and explained Dave's ill effects from the higher dose of Lipitor.

His cardiologist began to yell and scream stating "who cares about ill effects as Dave has coronary artery disease and he is diabetic."

As a specialist, we see our patients as that organ. To Dave's cardiologist, Dr. Brown, Dave is a heart and if he cannot walk, that is not Dr. Brown's problem. As far as Dr. Brown is concerned, Dave's heart is working fine with his recent medication adjustment. So, I returned to the exam room and let Dave know that Dr. Brown saved his life two years ago by inserting the stent into his coronary artery and Dave owes his life to Dr. Brown. However, as for our body's cellular function, Dr. Brown and I don't see eye to eye. He does not have the training or information to understand what happens to our cells with his treatment of the high dose statin.

Dave asked me to intervene and once we tapered his Lipitor dose down to 10 mg, he was able to walk up the stairs, think clearly, feel better, and he did not have any more aches and pains.

In this country we have the best medicine when it comes to acute illnesses such as heart attacks, strokes, trauma, etc. but we lack knowledge when it comes to chronic conditions. After all, insurance companies pay for illness and not wellness. Unsurprisingly, mainstream doctors wait till patients have acute diseases such as a heart attack, stroke, or diabetes with complications. Then they jump in and save lives and become heroes despite the fact that the patient may be incapacitated by his condition, lose his independence, be placed on many medications and perhaps even end up in a nursing home.

Somehow mainstream medical practitioners fail to consider that many medications have serious side effects. Wouldn't it be better if your doctor was able to foresee the illnesses approaching and give you a choice to change the path of your illness to the path of wellness, and make you your own hero?

If you think that is the way to go, consider seeking health care providers that practice functional medicine. There are many functional medicine doctors and providers practicing in your area. If you look for them, you will find them. Don't just trust any provider, mainstream or functional. Do your research and be proactive.

You need to take it one step further and interview your healthcare providers to make sure they are knowledgeable and caring. Always interview them and see if they listen to you.

Listening is an art and not everyone is blessed with this talent.

Make sure your health care providers don't get defensive when you question their knowledge. After all, you are putting your life in their hands. You want to make sure they are competent and they are open to any treatment that best suits you.

Medicine is not "one-size-fits-all". We are all made a little different and due to our genetic mutations, chemistry, and environmental factors, we respond differently to various treatments. Your healthcare providers should be open and willing to get you to an optimal state of health which may include medication, diet, exercise, nutrients, neurofeedback, pulsed electromagnetic field (PEMF), oxidative therapies, acupuncture, etc.

Your provider must be willing to learn how to help you even if it may not be their strong suit. I always have my patients challenge me. If I don't know the answer, I will let them know. I like to dig into research when confronted with a medical challenge and learn more about it to come up with an answer for them.

Being able to admit that "I don't know," as a physician, has made me more relatable to my patients. Wanting to learn about other treatments given by their other physicians, has made me investigate their health as a whole, and not just one organ; coincidentally, this shows my patients that I care about them, and they truly appreciate it.

Always encourage your health care providers to get your records from the last five years from all the other providers you have seen, and to review them. This shows that your doctor goes above and beyond to make sure other providers have not missed any serious health conditions or diagnosis.

I saw James as a new patient. He had intractable back pain and nothing seemed to help relieve it. I got a full history and ordered all his records from various physicians. I received volumes of chart information and reviewed them. I noticed a CT scan report of his lungs that showed a tumor in his left lung. Considering that James was an ex-smoker, I wanted to make sure his CT scan (from one year ago) was addressed appropriately. So, I invited James to my office and asked him what was done regarding the lung tumor noted in the CT scan of his lung. He appeared quite surprised and said "what tumor?" After reviewing the report, we gathered that his primary care physician (PCP) had retired. His PCP never saw the report. So James was lost in the shuffle of madness in medicine. I immediately ordered further studies along with a biopsy of his lung tumor. A week later James was in surgery for adenocarcinoma, a type of lung cancer. Today, he feels wonderful and has more energy than ever.

If you don't take charge of your health and don't hire the appropriate healthcare providers, you won't be aware of potential problems, and are setting yourself up for disasters in your health and wellness. Small signals in our bodies warn us of things that will become problematic in the future. There is no such thing as a "normal" symptom. Having a PCP that takes a functional approach to maintaining your health, as well as your active involvement in participating in that process, increases the likelihood of detecting the signals of a pending health issue. The sooner a problem is prevented from progressing the better, which will lead to a healthier and happier life.

EXERCISE

You are probably considering skipping this section because you heard so much about exercise, and you know you should do it, and yet you don't. I can promise you this is not the typical advice about exercise. First of all, your health is largely determined by three factors; what you put in your mouth, how you move your body, and how you handle stress. Food provides information to your DNA. How you move your body also positively impacts 60% of your genetic expression. If the benefits from exercise were in a pill, it would be the most popular pill on earth. Yet I often see patients who were so ill that even doing minimal exercise is very difficult for them. So I'm going to discuss the minimum effective dosage for exercise. Our ancestors did not spend hours in the gym; they were not running marathons, or half marathons, and they didn't have gym memberships.

The human body is designed to move. If you sit, you die, albeit slowly. Unfortunately, due to advancing technology, we are becoming increasingly inactive.

We see a lot of patients for medical weight loss. Since weight gain is a symptom of one or more medical problems, the program is designed to uncover the medical reasons for the weight gain. But in the first half we don't require them to do any exercise. Frankly, exercise is a very poor way to lose weight. Exercise is necessary to maintain weight and be healthy, but it is almost impossible to burn extra calories to get rid of excess fat. The amount of exercise needed would cause so many other metabolic problems, it would be counterproductive. We expect our patients to do 20 to 30 minutes of high quality exercise per week. I don't care what your circumstances, anyone can spare 20 to 30 minutes per week. The amount of exercise I ask of patients to do takes less time per day than it takes to get dressed to go to a gym, and it can be done in the bedroom.

First I need to explain about muscles. There are four types of muscle fibers:

Type 1 fibers	Active with low or no resistance
Type 2a fibers	Activated with increased resistance and type 1a fibers are not strong enough
Type 2x fibers	Activated with increased resistance and type 1a and 2a fibers are not strong enough
Type 2b fibers	Activated with near maximal effort, and type 1a, 2a, and 2x fibers are not strong enough

Suppose you move your arm to rest it on the table. Only type 1 fibers are firing. You could move it up and down a hundred times and still not work all of the muscles in your arm, because there is little to no resistance. If you picked up a 3 pound weight and moved your arm up and down, you would likely only be using type 1 and type 2a muscle fibers. Again, you are not exercising all of your muscle. The only way to completely exercise all four of the muscle fibers is to do high resistance, and to do high resistance you cannot do high repetitions. Instead of lifting weights where you need to do three sets of 20 repetitions, you should lift the weight that you can lift three times, but not more than five times. If you can lift the weight more than five times, the weight is too light. If you do a set of 20 repetitions, most of them aren't doing anything other than making the first three types of fibers tire out, so that you will finally be straining on the final lifts so the type 2b fibers will be activated.

The type 2b fibers have greater force but less endurance; but by working them, you are working all four muscle fiber types. You can actually exercise less, but derive more benefit from the shorter workouts. Type 2b muscle fibers need at least six days to recover from the exercise.

If you exercise on a regular basis and suffer from a stroke years later, you are more likely to recover with little to no permanent damage. Whereas, if you lived an inactive and sedentary life, the same exact stroke will cause a great deal of disability. This is because exercise causes neuron's dendrites, which are root-like structures of brain cells, to grow long and bypass the affected area. But if you don't exercise, your dendrites will be short and will not bypass the area affected by the stroke, and thus, they will be unable to communicate with the adjacent neurons in that affected area, leading to disability.

When you exercise, you increase oxygenation to every tissue and cell in your body, which in turn, will increase your cells' oxygen processing capacity and you feel rejuvenated, even if it is five minutes of exercise a day. The good news is you have control over your movements.

Moving certain muscles are necessary for you to reach the hormonal requirements for your body's optimum function.

Your nutrition and diet play a huge role in your longevity.

A major dietary toxin is sugar. We consume over 150 pounds of sugar a year on average; some consume even more than this. If you read food labels, you can still miss hidden sugars in those processed foods.

In women, fructose is processed by their liver; in men, it's processed by both their sperm and liver. Are you wondering why over the years you have lost your waist line? If so, take a close look at your diet. Numerous research articles by Dr. Lustig at UCSF regarding sugar and its many health hazards are available on this subject.

Why do you think diabetics whose condition is poorly controlled can become blind, suffer amputated toes and limbs, have kidney failure requiring dialysis, and have early onset heart attacks and strokes?

The answer is sugar!

As previously mentioned, the new name for Alzheimer's disease is now diabetes type III. Sugar can cross the filter at the base of our brain called blood-brain barrier. This filter's function is to keep toxins from entering the brain so that there won't be insults to your brain cells. However, sugar crosses through the blood-brain barrier, enters the neurons or brain cells and attacks them. Over time you will have lost enough neurons that you look at your loved ones and say "Who are you people"?

So, if you are concerned about losing your independence 10 to 15 years down the road, stop eating sugar now. A common myth is that eating fruits, grains, starches and drinking wine are good for you. These items are loaded with sugar and can cause a myriad of health problems. The response center in the brain for sugar is on the same site as it is for cocaine and heroin. So, naturally, when you attempt to avoid sugar, your body will crave it and may even go through withdrawals which may take a month or more to overcome. You need to see your functional medicine doctor, nutritionist, chiropractor, naturopathic doctor, acupuncturist, etc. to help you clean up your diet.

At our clinic we use a seven-day blood sugar monitor to get accurate information on our patient's blood sugar readings. This method can help screen our patients for diabetes early on so that our patients can change their path of illness to the path of wellness.

Other major unhealthy foods are grains, especially grains that contain gluten. Dr. William Davis, the author of "Wheat Belly", Dr. Perlmutter, the author of "Grain Brain", and Dr. Fasano's (a celiac disease expert) have written extensively on gluten as a culprit for many health conditions.

Next in the list of foods to avoid is dairy. Yes, I am taking your joy away. So, no cheese or crackers. This is when my patients like me less. But after one month they come back and tell me they like me more. It's amazing how much energy people get when they quit grains, sugars and dairy. You can still have your cheese and crackers, but they need to be grain-and dairy-free. Those options are available in many health food stores and/or online.

Gluten-free does not equal grain free. This has been a common misconception with over 30,000 patients that I have treated. Always read labels, because what you assume is safe may be harmful to your cells.

Try to avoid corn and GMO foods. Eat grass-fed meats and free-range chicken. Avoid farmed salmon or seafood that may contain a high mercury load.

PROBIOTICS

We have over one hundred trillion best friends that live within our body. These nice creatures reside mostly in our gut and protect us against many maladies. They get rid of toxins, decrease your bad cholesterol, increase your immune system, improve your mood and sleep, help with bone formation, protect your brain cells, help heal your gastrointestinal lining, decrease inflammation, help with fat loss, and many more functions.

Did you know that 70% of your immune system is housed in your gut? Did you also know that 90% of your serotonin receptors are in your gut? This is why you get a stomach ache or diarrhea or butterflies when you're anxious. Your gut is known to be your second brain and there is a gut-brain connection in our body. Thus, ingesting probiotics, which add the "good guys" to our gut helps with many cognitive functions. Unfortunately, due to the antibiotic era and lack of fiber in our diet, we are killing our healthy gut bacteria and allowing other unhealthy creatures to grow and occupy our gastrointestinal tract causing inflammation and leading to many health problems.

Intermittent fasting and calorie restriction also help with longevity. Periodic fasting protects neurons against many insults such as strokes, Parkinson's disease, and Alzheimer's disease. Intermittent fasting and caloric restriction cause mild stress to systems, leading to an increases in BDNF (brain derived neuro- tropic factor), a protein that prevents stressed neurons from dying.

Chapter Six

SLEEP

We cannot function without a good night's sleep. Our sleep cycle has a pattern known as circadian rhythm. There are different hormones and neurotransmitters that are involved with our sleep cycles. Once you sleep, you enter a light sleep phase followed by deep sleep phase and then REM sleep phase, known as the dream phase. A full sleep cycle lasts approximately ninety minutes and will repeat itself multiple times throughout the night.

Sleep is a major part of our longevity. It affects our mood, memory, attention, cognitive functions, decision-making, immune system, stress hormones and our weight. Sleep allows the body and mind to rest, replenish and repair. During sleep, our body produces hormones that help us with our vitality. Melatonin is a hormone produced by the pineal gland in our brain and is synthesized and released into our bloodstream in the presence of darkness. Any light will signal the brain to hold off on making and releasing melatonin. Even if you cover your eyes, you cannot fool your body. During deep sleep we release melatonin which helps us remain asleep. On the contrary, your melatonin levels drop significantly in presence of light and you wake up. I had a blind patient, Joanne, who was enrolled in my weight loss program. Her husband used to drive her for hours to see me every two weeks. She was following the program religiously and losing weight accordingly. One day during her visit, we noted that she had not lost any weight since her previous visit two weeks earlier. Joanne was quite disappointed. I asked her many questions trying to find out why her weight loss had stalled.

"Joanne, have you changed your diet?" "No", she replied.

"Have you changed your physical activity levels?" "No" she replied.

"Have you started a new medication or over-the-counter drugs or supplements?" "No" she replied.

"Have you been under stress recently?" "No" she replied.

"Have you been traveling?" No" she replied.

"Have you been celebrating any special occasions?" "No" she replied.

"Have you been using a night light in your bedroom?" Yes! she replied.

"How long have you been using the nightlight?" She answered, "Approximately 10 days, Dr. Shaban."

"This is the reason why you have not lost weight over the last two weeks."

"Dr. Shaban, you do realize that I am blind?" I smiled and said "I know, but your skin has "eyes" and can detect light which signals your brain to see the light. This prohibits your melatonin from synthesizing and prevents you from getting a good night sleep." Apparently, Joanne's husband had left town for 10 days while he was on a work trip. Joanne's niece had stayed with her during that time and placed the nightlight in Joanne's bedroom so that she could check up on Joanne during the night. Once Joanne removed the nightlight, she began to lose weight again and eventually reached her goal. The explanation for her outcome is because light affects the skin which in turn, messages the brain to avoid releasing melatonin.

It is best to take all of the electronics out of your bedroom, remove the lights, be sure to have a comfortable mattress and bedding, avoid drinking excessive water before bedtime, avoid working on any projects in bed and avoid stimulants such as caffeine. If you are on a diuretic, stimulant medications, steroids or thyroid medication, make sure to take them early in the morning as they can affect your sleep.

Some medications can cause insomnia. These include but are not limited to SSRIs such as Prozac and Zoloft,

Parkinson medications, amphetamine derived medications, anti-seizure medications, decongestants, diuretics, and some cholesterol-lowering medications.

If you are under a great deal of stress and feel anxious, you may have a hard time falling asleep. Deep breathing exercises and meditation can help decrease anxiety levels and help you sleep. There are some devices that help with balancing your autonomic nervous system (sympathetic and parasympathetic nervous system) and can help you sleep better. I use Inner Balance (Heart Math) in my practice to help my patients with anxiety and insomnia. They can use the app on their smartphone and practice their deep breathing exercises at any time. This eliminates any excuses patients may have about this exercise.

If you, or your partner snore or stop breathing during the night, you need to be evaluated for sleep apnea or other sleep disorders. A polysomnogram is used to evaluate sleep disorders. It checks airflow, blood oxygen levels, brain activities, eye movements, hearts rate, blood pressure, snoring events, and chest movement to see if there is any effort with breathing.

I had a 68-year-old gentleman, 'Mr. Smith', in my practice and during my initial evaluation I heard a murmur (abnormal heart sound). I obtained an echocardiogram which showed heart changes compatible with long-standing hypertension (HTN). When I reviewed his echocardiogram results and asked him how long he had suffered from HTN, he was quite upset and said he took pride in his blood pressure always being normal. He had always been told by all of his physicians that his blood pressure was mostly 110/60 and was reassured that his blood pressure was that of a 20-year-old's and he was reassured that he was not at risk for heart attack or stroke.

First and foremost, a blood pressure reading at your doctor's office can be very misleading. If your blood pressure is high at that moment in the office, does it mean that you suffer from HTN? Could you have been anxious or had caffeine 15 minutes before your blood pressure check? If your blood pressure is low at that moment, does that make you a normotensive person? The answer to these questions are "not necessarily".

Back to my patient, Mr. Smith. I placed him on a 24 hour blood pressure monitor. This device gives me information on numerous blood pressure readings within a 24-hour period. The following day, when he returned the device, I noted his blood pressure was 110/60 all day; however within 45 minutes after he fell asleep, his blood pressure rose to 220/120, 180/110, 240/100, etc. and once he woke up, his blood pressure was back to 110/60 again.

Mr. Smith would be an example of a person who could have had a major heart attack or stroke during his sleep. Obviously, none of his physicians would have picked up this abnormality without doing the 24-hour pressure monitor. When I reviewed his blood pressure report with him, he asked what could be the cause of his nocturnal HTN. I explained he could be suffering from sleep apnea. Once again, he became defensive and said he took pride in being in shape, and indeed he appeared quite fit and lean. It is a myth to think if you aren't overweight or obese, you won't have sleep apnea.

I have diagnosed patients with sleep apnea who have been quite lean. Our next venture with Mr. Smith was to send him home with a portable diagnostic device which monitors the patient's breathing, sleep patterns, oxygenation, heart rate, etc.

Sure enough, Mr. Smith's sleep apnea test showed severe sleep apnea. Once we addressed his sleep apnea with a dental device (since the patient did not prefer CPAP), his 24-hour blood pressure monitor showed normal blood pressure readings throughout the night. Interestingly, Mr. Smith's agitation which was a symptom of hypoxemia (low blood oxygen), was resolved and he became a very pleasant patient.

Mr. Smith could have been a victim of an unrecognized health condition that may have very well led to a major stroke, heart attack, debilitation, or death. When your doctor diagnoses you with a health condition or places you on a medication, you should be proactive; study and research your health condition, and always seek a second opinion from a non-conventional physician or healthcare professional.

This is only one example out of many where a life-threatening condition was discovered through functional medicine that prevented the patient having to pay the consequence of a major or fatal condition.

Sometimes, I tell my patients to eat a small, balanced snack before bedtime since in some patients low blood sugar can trigger cortisol levels to increase during the night disturbing their sleep.

HEAVY METALS

Heavy metals such as aluminum, mercury, and lead are neurotoxic and can cause insomnia. These metals can cause many central nervous system and peripheral nervous system disturbances leading to neuropathy or other kinds of pain that can interfere with your sleep. Have your functional medicine provider check you for heavy metals and help you eliminate them from your system.

There are many ways you can check for heavy metals. Mainstream physicians use blood or urine samples to detect heavy metals. These tests will not show any abnormalities since heavy metals tend to attach themselves to the tissues and since they are not in the bloodstream, they won't be in the urine as the kidneys filter what is in our circulatory system. Most mainstream doctors rely on blood or urine and advise the patient that they don't have elevated lead, mercury, etc. levels. Therefore heavy metals may not be detected in patients who can easily then be misdiagnosed.

Suppose you eat some tuna that has mercury in it. Blood tests show elevated mercury for days but within a week the mercury levels will be back to the level before you ate the fish. One of two things will have happened. Either your body will have excreted the mercury, or the mercury will have been absorbed into your own tissue. If it was absorbed into your tissue, we have no way of assessing your total body burden of heavy metals.

At my office, we use a six-hour urine test. Patients are told to avoid seafood for a week. When they wake up they collect the first morning urine sample followed by taking two different chelating agents; their urine is then collected at intervals for the next six hours.

If left untreated, the heavy metals can cause a great deal of health issues. They can cause plaque formation in arteries, neuropathy, fatigue problems, bone loss such as osteopenia or osteoporosis, decrease sense of touch, hearing, vision, produce a metallic taste in the mouth, cause headaches, pre-hypertension, irritability, insomnia, tremors, balance issues, anemia, psychotic and manic behaviors, kidney failure, and immune suppression leading to various cancers. They can also lead to autoimmune disorders. In children, it can cause developmental disorders and mental illness. You may ask,"How do I get heavy metals?" These agents are seen in our environment. For instance, the common exposures to mercury are from dental amalgams or seafood consumption. Many mainstream dentists, like mainstream physicians, are not knowledgeable about these metals and may try to convince you that metals are harmless. Heavy metals compete with other detoxification pathways, such as those used to eliminate plastics. Your body has a limited capacity to eliminate toxins from the body every day. Reducing your daily total body burden of toxins is essential.

If your dentist doesn't acknowledge that heavy metals can cause health issues, seek an integrative dentist who is knowledgeable to keep you from becoming chronically ill. Fortunately, there are major efforts in place to ban mercury fillings worldwide. The USA is, of course, lagging behind most other nations.

As you can see, getting a false negative blood or urine test be quite harmful to you if you have elevated levels of heavy metals in your tissue. For some patients, heavy metals are the main cause of their symptoms. The sooner you get these agents out of your system, the less damage will occur and the faster you will recover. Thus, you can prevent many future illnesses if you see a provider who can evaluate you appropriately.

Another cause of insomnia is consuming high-fat foods at bedtime. I tell my patients to eat the high-fat foods hours before bedtime to assure proper digestion. If you have had gallbladder surgery, you may not be able to digest fats and thus be unable to absorb them. You may think that it is beneficial if you don't absorb fats. However, fats are great for our health. By that I mean good fats and not trans-fats. Trans-fats are found in hydrogenated oils, as well as in all vegetable oils, especially soybean and canola oil. Soybean and canola oils are found in virtually all processed foods and in most restaurants.

Our brains are mostly water, but by dry weight, the brain is made of mostly fat and cholesterol. Yes, we are all "fat heads". Every cell in our body has a cell membrane, which is made of phospholipids. The cells interact with each other by passing messages through their cell membranes. If you do not eat or absorb enough healthy fats, your cell membrane will stiffen and your cell-to-cell communication will be impaired.

Once you consume fat and it enters your intestines, bile is released from your gallbladder. The bile acts like a soap to emulsify and the enzymes then break down the fats to be absorbed.

Sometimes, I tell my patients to eat a small, balanced snack before bedtime since in some patients low blood sugar can trigger cortisol levels to increase during the night disturbing their sleep.

Alcohol consumed before bedtime will reduce rapid eye movement (REM) sleep. The more alcohol you consume, the more likely you will not have restful sleep.

Restless leg syndrome is another condition that can affect your sleep quality. If you cannot control your limbs from jerking during the night, you need to discuss this with your healthcare provider and try to find the underlying cause of your condition. This condition can be due to nutrient deficiencies or neurological conditions.

If you are experiencing hot flashes or night sweats, you need to be evaluated for hormonal imbalance and/or other serious health conditions such as lymphomas or systemic infections.

Sometimes napping has been shown to help my patients with recharging. These naps are usually 10 to 30 minutes in length and are taken between 2-4 PM.

Melatonin

Melatonin is now considered to be the most potent antiaging hormone. In this day and age, we are aging rapidly as we are not producing enough melatonin and other hormones due to our lifestyle and lack of appropriate amount and quality of sleep.

Melatonin in high doses, has an anticancer action. Melatonin is used to help with insomnia, jetlag, seasonal affective disorder, shift workers, tinnitus and much more.

Sleep deprivation affects the hippocampus in a negative manner. This is the center of the brain that holds pleasant memories. People with insomnia have lasting negative and gloomy memories.

Growth hormone production is partly dependent on sleep duration, timing and quality. It helps with our growth, bone and muscle formation, sugar and fat metabolism and elevates energy levels.

During sleep, our body and cells rejuvenate. Our brain's oligodendrites get to work and act as garbage trucks, cleaning the trash left behind in our brain that cause brain fog. Do you wake up with a fuzzy brain? If so, have your health care provider look for sleep disorders. You must wake up with a clear mind if you sleep well through the night. The recommended sleep hours are 11 PM to 7 AM. For best results, you need to sleep approximately eight hours a night. If you are a shift worker, you are likely having major hormonal imbalances and are at risk of many health conditions. You can try to avoid the health problems as a shift worker if you sleep during the day and are up all night consistently. But, if you alter your sleep hours on your days off, your hormones remain off tune and your music will not sound pleasant and as a result you won't feel well.

Did you know your peak fat-burning time occurs while you are asleep? It will be hard to lose weight or maintain your weight loss if you do not get your eight hours of sleep per night.

Also, you need to sleep in a completely dark room. Any light, will send a signal to your brain to wake up. Your skin has "eyes". It detects light and sends a message to your brain to stop producing melatonin. Melatonin is released when it is nighttime or during complete darkness. There is communication between your skin and your brain. Darkness causes your skin to communicate with your brain to release melatonin so that you can remain asleep; and during daytime, or with presence of any light, your skin signals your brain to stop the melatonin release so that you can wake up. Therefore, any light in your room such as your iPhone, alarm clock, or nightlight can interfere with this process and lead to hormonal imbalances. Sometimes a low dose of melatonin taken orally can help with insomnia. You need to talk to your functional medicine provider to see if you are a suitable candidate.

Progesterone is another hormone that helps you remain asleep. During perimenopause and menopause our progesterone levels decline which, in turn, causes insomnia and anxiety. Therefore, balancing your hormones will improve your sleep.

There are also certain nutrients such as magnesium, certain herbs such as threonine, holy basil and other adrenal support remedies, valerian root and 5-HTP that may also help improve insomnia. These nutrients need to be purchased from a reputable nutraceutical company.

Meditation and deep breathing techniques can help with balancing your autonomic nervous system. Your sympathetic nervous system is your fight or flight response system and your parasympathetic nervous system is your rest and digest system. These two systems are responsible for the autonomic functions of your body, which are bodily functions that you should not be aware of on regular basis. For instance, your heart rate, bowel movement, breathing etc. If you are in sympathetic overload, you will have difficulty sleeping. Addressing your autonomic nervous system can help with insomnia. This is explained in more detail in the section on stress.

Cortisol is your stress hormone and is released in a rhythmic pattern. In the morning you should have the most amount of cortisol and as the day goes by, your levels should drop to the lowest amount before your sleep. If this pattern is disturbed, you will have a difficult time sleeping. Elevated cortisol levels tend to increase your insulin levels which will hold on to every fat cell, making your weight loss attempts unsuccessful. It is important to address your stress so that you can get a good night's sleep.

Chapter Seven
⤳ **STEP 7** ⤳

STRESS

S tress is one of the most destructive forces that acts on our body in our modern world. Stress is linked to every chronic illness, and is one of the main root causes of every condition we treat. If you are being chased by a tiger, you will either outrun it, or you will not. Either way, your stress will be over quickly. If you THINK you are being chased by a tiger, the exact same physiological changes occur in your body: Adrenalin and cortisol are released into the blood, your pupils dilate, your blood pressure and pulse rate increase. However, stress is inevitable with our current lifestyles.

Our emotional, mental, social and behavioral factors will directly affect our physical health. Stress is the culprit for many health problems. Unless you learn to handle your stress, it will destroy you. Stress affects every organ in our body; it causes an increase in cortisol hormone levels leading to hormonal imbalance. Stress causes the negative thoughts to override the positive thoughts and leads to the unhappy peptide release, causing negative events to spin out of control. The elevated cortisol will hold onto insulin, making you insulin resistant, which in turn holds onto your fat cells leading to weight gain despite proper diet and exercise. Stress makes you vulnerable to infections and cancer by suppressing your immune system.

Stress interferes with all your other hormonal imbalances and leads to aging skin; it affects your thyroid hormone, leads to memory loss and many other health issues. Your autonomic nervous system will also be affected by your stress, leading to sympathetic nervous system over activity which affects your heart, gastrointestinal tract, and other organs.

Stress interferes with the balance between your neurotransmitters, thus leading to insomnia, depression and anxiety.

As you can see by now, we are not made up of one organ or one system. Every cell is affected positively or negatively by these seven basic concepts. When your cardiologist places you on cholesterol medication in hopes to regulate your cholesterol, your body becomes depleted of multiple essential nutrients which in turn leads to hormonal imbalance and all the other health problems. When people are not stressed they tend to start eating healthier and exercising and keeping up with their healthy lifestyle.

How Does a Person De-stress?

Let's focus on deep breathing. When done correctly, you can decrease your cortisol levels by 50%. How do you know if you are breathing deeply enough to decrease your cortisol levels? You would need to look into devices such as Inner Balance (Heart Math). This is a well-researched device with a great deal of scientific data. You can install it on your computer or smartphone. This device shows a circular image on the screen that changes color with every breath you take; the goal is to keep your breathing so that the circle remains green. The Mayo Clinic has been using this device for pain management. If you can't measure it, you can't manage it. Therefore, it is best to have a device that will confirm your accurate breathing techniques.

Hugs

Seven hugs a day will increase the hormone oxytocin, also known as the love hormone, or cuddle hormone. Oxytocin is released from the posterior pituitary gland in your brain. This hormone is needed for de-stressing. Oxytocin also helps people bond socially. This is the hormone that promotes the mother-child bonding. Even playing with your pet will increase your oxytocin levels. Oxytocin affects your emotions, cognition, and social behavior.

LAUGHTER

Laughter is the best medication to help with stress reduction. Laughter decreases the stress hormone and increases immunity, thus improving your resistance to infections and cancer. Laughter triggers the release of endorphins, the body's natural feel-good chemicals. Endorphins promote an overall sense of well-being and can help with pain relief. Thus, laughter is a powerful antidote to stress, pain and conflict. Laughter enhances oxygen intake, relaxes muscles throughout our bodies, relieves pain, improves alertness, memory and creativity, improves sleep and produces a general sense of well-being.

Other means of stress relief may include:

- Talking to someone you trust
- Being in the present moment
- Massage
- Singing/listening to music/playing a musical instrument
- Dancing
- Coloring/drawing/painting
- Breathing
- Moving your body (chi gong, Tai chi)
- Hot baths

- Crying
- Essential oils
- Meditation
- Yoga
- Forgiveness
- Love
- Prayer/Faith/spirituality
- Good support system
- Being grateful
- Exercising
- Gardening
- Grounding/walking barefoot 30 minutes a day
- Hanging around positive people
- Intimacy/touching/kissing
- Connecting with people
- Time management/avoiding last minute deadlines
- Watching a funny movie
- Acknowledging your successes and your failures
- Emotional freedom techniques/tapping
- Asking for help/talking to a friend, family member or a therapist
- Being passionate

- Snuggling with your loved ones and your pet
- PMF
- Visualization
- Reading books that make you feel good
- Facing your fears
- Decreasing your expectations
- Stress management can be extremely helpful if you make it a daily part of your lifestyle

Chapter Eight

Platelet Rich Plasma Joint and Soft Tissue Injections

Another popular procedure in my clinic is platelet rich plasma (PRP). We use this procedure as an alternative option to surgery for joint injections, facial rejuvenation, breast lift, O-shot and P-shot. Mainstream medicine offers anti-inflammatory and pain medications, cortisone shots, hyaluronic acid injections, arthroscopic surgeries, and major joint or ligament and tendon surgical repairs, to address conditions such as osteoarthritis of shoulders, rotator cuff tears, osteoarthritis of elbows, wrists, hands, hips, knees, ankles and feet.

Anti-inflammatory and pain medications have side effects that include constipation, bowel impaction, gastrointestinal ulcerations and bleeding, addiction to narcotics, increase risk of falls and injuries, heart disease and hypertension.

Patients on narcotic medications will also be unable to drive after surgery and are at risk for addiction.

A cortisone shot is only a temporary pain relief and can weaken the tendon and cause more problems.

Arthroscopic surgery will have a longer recovery time and involves more risks than PRP as far as infection and wound healing.

Surgery can have multiple complications:

These include complication due to anesthesia, poor wound healing, infection, intraoperative device failure, long recovery (few weeks), postoperative blood clot complications such as deep venous thrombosis (DVT) or pulmonary embolism (PE), time lost from work, loss of independence during the time of recovery, and death.

PRP has been researched since the 1970s but did not receive much publicity until the recent years. PRP is an in office procedure that relieves the pain, repairs and treats injured tissues. There is no use of general or systemic anesthesia or a hospital stay.

The majority of my patients return to work the same day and can drive into and out of my clinic.

The effectiveness of PRP depends on the patient's health status. The healthier the patient the better the response will be with this procedure. There is no risk involved as we use the patient's own blood.

PRP procedure is quite simple and painless with rapid recovery period. There is no downtime.

Prior to PRP, we obtain the patient's health history, examine the patient and review any imaging available. The patient is advised to refrain from certain blood thinners and supplements. Then the patient's blood is drawn and spun in a special centrifuge. The platelet rich plasma is then separated and prepared for injection. The area to be injected is then cleaned and topical anesthetic is used prior to PRP injection into the affected joint or tissue.

The entire procedure takes less than one hour and the patient is advised to take it easy with no strenuous activities for one to three days.

Most of my patients do not require any medication prior to this procedure. I advise my patients to avoid taking any anti-inflammatory medications pre-and-post procedure since it will interfere with optimum PRP response. I prefer use of heat over cold packs after the treatment.

The PRP stimulates a series of biologic responses which aids in the healing process. Therefore, taking anti-inflammatory medications will interfere with this process.

Platelets are a normal component of our blood and release growth factors and other proteins that stimulate tissue regeneration, thus promote healing. PRP has up to nine times the concentration of platelets found in our blood.

Post procedure, patients will note a decrease in pain, improvement in the joint function, and regeneration of newly formed tissues seen on follow-up imaging.

It may take up to three months for patients to achieve these results. I refer my patients to physical therapy to help them strengthen the affected muscles and joints and to teach correct movements to maintain their strength and flexibility.

I use PRP to treat osteoarthritis of various joints, ACL injuries, ankle and elbow injuries and sprains, rotator cuff tears, TMJ and trigger fingers. If a patient's injury is severe, I may add bone marrow stem cells aspirated from their hip bone, prolozone therapy, or even amniotic fluid which has been obtained from a full-term newborn.

Although most of my patients will need one treatment, some may need up to three treatments to get the desired response.

I also use PRP for breast augmentation, facelift and facial rejuvenation, O-shot and P-shot.

Always search other options when you are told surgery is your option.

I have patients with severe urinary issues such as urinary incontinence which is debilitating to them and affects their social life. I have heard of patients giving up jogging, yoga, going to the gym, and other activities simply because they leak urine with any physical activities. Other women have told me they aren't as intimate with their partners because they smell like urine. Some women suffer from urinary urgency and their life is consumed by their bladder issues. One of my patients, "Leslie", came to me stating her marriage is at stake. Due to her urinary frequency, she was utilizing the restroom every 15 minutes. This had caused disturbances in her life. Her husband wouldn't sit by her since it was too disturbing to him. He would not eat at the same table, watch movies or go anyplace with her. Leaving the house to go to any appointment was a chore for Leslie as she would have to map out her drive to and from any point since she needed access to a restroom on her route. She had tried multiple medications but was unable to tolerate them due to severe side effects such as severe mouth dryness. Leslie saw me on a Friday and received her O-shot.

She returned the following Monday demanding to see me. My staff notified me of her unexpected visit and I asked them to get Leslie into a room. I was expecting to hear that the shot did not work and I was ready to remind her that it can take up to two months to see results. Instead as I walked in to the room, she gave me a great big hug and cried. I just held her in my arms until she finally settled down and spoke.

"When I left your office on Friday night, I didn't urinate for four hours and I thought it was all psychological. But over the weekend, I managed to urinate as I used to in my 20s and 30s. My husband and I cried all weekend in hopes that our lives will return to somewhat normal again. He actually held me all weekend and this morning he booked us a cruise. I cannot thank you enough for giving me my life back". We sure take our health for granted. Don't we?

The O-shot is a procedure that uses platelet rich plasma from your own blood, and is then concentrated and injected into the clitoris and vagina. This stimulates and rejuvenates the areas injected. It helps with urinary incontinence, increases libido (sex drive), helps with painful sex, as well as itching and burning sensation in the vagina due to dryness. The O-shot improves sexual sensations leading to improved orgasm. This is an in-office procedure and the effects last about one year. We apply numbing cream to the areas we plan to inject. The procedure takes about one hour and the patient can drive herself out of the office. We have our patients fill out a questionnaire as they are numbing. Their blood is drawn and spun in a specific centrifuge to concentrate their platelet rich plasma (PRP). Once the PRP is available, the procedure takes less than 15 minutes. Patients may feel some pressure just as they do with a Pap smear. There is no pain involved. There are no restrictions with their activities after the procedure. However, I recommend my patients avoid bicycling or horseback riding for one week after the procedure as it may be uncomfortable. They can have intercourse immediately post-procedure. They may see some spotting the day of their O-shot procedure which is not unusual. Once patients receive their O-shot, they are advised to avoid any anti-inflammatory medications or steroids for approximately one month. When PRP is injected, it creates an inflammatory reaction which in turn will call in the patient's own stem cells to navigate to the injected areas and initiate the healing process. Taking anti-inflammatory drugs will interfere with the inflammation process needed for the O-shot to work optimally. I encourage my patients to perform pelvic floor exercises to help strengthen pelvis tissue and make their O-shot last longer. This procedure was invented by Dr. Charles Runnels, MD and it has become one of the most popular procedures done in our clinic. One of my patients who received the O-shot told me she was unable to hold her urine when she got out of bed in the mornings. She had refrained from sexual intercourse as she did not want to share this experience with anyone to witness. She told me the O-shot has changed her life and she is now able to be intimate once again after many years. Another patient told me she can now sleep through the night after receiving the O-shot. Since her sleep has improved, her energy, mood, and her overall health has improved significantly. Another one of my patients had suffered from a condition called lichen sclerosis. She tells me the O-shot has cured her lichen sclerosis. It is so gratifying to make a significant difference in so many women's lives by just a simple in office procedure. Unfortunately, many physicians are unaware of this option for their patients. As a result, these patients seek medication or surgical options with possible risks, complications and side effects.

Another procedure unknown to so many is the P-shot. The P-shot is done by drawing blood from our male patients and separating the growth factors and injecting it to their genital region. This procedure will improve libido, erection, ejaculation, and will help with increasing penile size. For many men, love is expressed by sexual performance. For most women, love is more emotional. Being held, caressed and being told how beautiful they look is what a woman may need to feel loved, wanted and even aroused. I have male patients who tell me as they have aged, they have noticed a loss of volume in their genital region and ask what, if anything, can be done about it.

We live in a world where technology has become so advanced that a single shot from your own blood can improve this concern and help these gentlemen be able to feel confident once again. Of course, we always address all the other health issues including vascular, hormonal, nitric oxide levels, oxygenation, etc. to get them to reach their destination. The P-shot uses the patient's own blood and then it is spun in a special centrifuge. PRP and growth factors are extracted. The genital region is numbed using topical numbing cream. The PRP is then injected into the male genitalia and it is completely painless. I have not had any patient complain of discomfort during or after the procedure. The procedure takes less than one hour and they can drive themselves out of the office. They are given and advised to use a pump 10 minutes per day for two months. Men need two P-shots, 4 to 6 weeks apart. They are advised to avoid any anti-inflammatory medications or steroids for two months. This procedure lasts about one year with great satisfaction to our male patients and their partners.

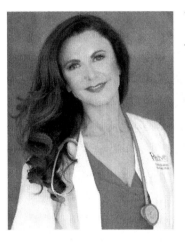

Dr. Shaban is triple board-certified in internal medicine, geriatrics and functional medicine and certified in metabolic cardiology, bioidentical hormone replacement therapy, bone marrow stem cell therapy, O-shots, P-shots and cosmetic procedures. She uses cutting-edge technology in her clinic including bone marrow stem cell therapy, oxidative therapy, IV nutritional therapy, platelet-rich plasma and multiple computerized devices to predict illnesses years in advance and give her patients a choice to change their path to wellness.